EMBRACE THE REFRESH:

A HOLISTIC APPROACH TO DRY EYE SOLUTIONS

DR. MELISSA P. NELSON

All rights reserved. No part of this publication may be reproduced, distributed, or transmitted in any form or by any means, including photocopying, recording, or other electronic or mechanical methods, without the prior written permission of the publisher, except in the case of brief quotations embodied in critical reviews and certain other noncommercial uses permitted by copyright law.

Copyright © Dr. Melissa P. Nelson, 2023.

TABLE OF CONTENTS

INTRODUCTION

Welcome to "Embrace the Refresh: A Holistic Approach to Dry Eye Solutions." In this book, we invite you to embark on a transformative journey towards optimal eye health and lasting relief from dry eye discomfort. If you've ever experienced the irritation, grittiness, or blurry vision associated with dry eye, you know how crucial it is to find effective solutions that address not just the symptoms but the underlying causes.

Dry eye is a prevalent and multifaceted condition that affects millions of individuals worldwide. Beyond the conventional remedies, we believe that a holistic approach is the key to unlocking the true potential for healing and rejuvenation. In these pages, we'll delve into the interconnectedness of our physical, emotional, and environmental well-being, discovering how they converge to impact the health of our precious eyes.

Our journey begins with a comprehensive understanding of dry eye syndrome – its triggers, variations, and the far-reaching consequences it can have on our overall eye health. We'll explore the intricate workings of our eyes, demystifying the underlying factors that contribute to dry eye, and equipping you with the knowledge to make informed decisions about your eye care.

Beyond the physical aspects, we will embrace the often-overlooked emotional dimension of dry eye. Stress, anxiety, and lifestyle choices all play a significant role in our ocular comfort. By addressing the mind-body connection, we'll discover how holistic practices, stress reduction techniques, and lifestyle adjustments can enhance our eye health and overall well-being.

Fueling our bodies with the right nutrients is essential for optimal eye function. In these pages, we'll explore a cornucopia of eye-friendly foods and supplements that nourish our eyes from the inside out, supporting tear production and promoting eye moisture.

But it's not just about what we consume; it's also about how we interact with our environment. We'll uncover the impact of hydration, proper eye hygiene, and environmental factors on dry eye discomfort, empowering you to make meaningful changes that lead to relief.

As we progress, we'll uncover the potential of herbal remedies, compresses, and aromatherapy as natural allies in our dry eye journey. Together, we'll explore the exciting realm of emerging treatments and advanced solutions for severe dry eye cases, staying at the forefront of eye care innovation.

To empower you further, we'll guide you in crafting your personalized dry eye action plan. We'll set goals, track progress, and embrace the refreshment of a holistic approach that will not only alleviate your current symptoms but also safeguard your eye health for the long term.

In "Embrace the Refresh," you'll find a harmonious fusion of evidence-based research, practical advice, and a compassionate understanding of the challenges faced by those seeking relief from dry eye. Our aim is to help you become the steward of your own eye health, embracing the refreshment of a vibrant, comfortable, and rejuvenated perspective on life.

So, come along on this transformative journey, and let's embark on a holistic approach to dry eye solutions. Together, we'll unveil the power of self-care, nourishment, and rejuvenation, welcoming the refreshing comfort that awaits us at the heart of holistic eye health.

CHAPTER 1: UNDERSTANDING DRY EYE

Dry eye is a common ocular condition characterized by an imbalance in the quantity or quality of tears, leading to an insufficient lubrication and nourishment of the eyes. Tears play a crucial role in maintaining eye health by providing a smooth surface for clear vision, protecting against infections, and nourishing the ocular tissues.

What Is Dry Eye Syndrome?

Dry eye syndrome, also known as keratoconjunctivitis sicca, is a common and multifaceted ocular condition that affects millions of people worldwide. At its core, dry eye syndrome occurs when there is an imbalance in the quantity or quality of tears produced by the eyes, leading to an insufficient lubrication and nourishment of the ocular surface.

Tears play a vital role in maintaining the health and function of the eyes. They are composed of a complex combination of water, oils, mucus, and specialized proteins, each serving a unique purpose. The watery component, produced by the lacrimal glands, helps to cleanse and hydrate the eyes, while the oil produced by the meibomian glands forms a protective layer on the tear film, reducing evaporation.

Mucus, generated by the goblet cells, aids in distributing tears evenly across the surface of the eye.

When there is an inadequate production of tears, or the balance of these components is disrupted, the tear film becomes unstable. This can result in a range of uncomfortable symptoms, including dryness, grittiness, burning sensations, and occasional excessive tearing as the body attempts to compensate for the lack of proper lubrication.

Causes And Risk Factors

The causes and risk factors of dry eye syndrome are multifaceted and can vary from person to person. Understanding these underlying factors is essential in effectively managing and treating the condition. Below are some common causes and risk factors associated with dry eye syndrome:

Environmental Factors: Exposure to dry and windy climates, air conditioning, and indoor heating can accelerate tear evaporation and contribute to dry eye symptoms. Additionally, spending prolonged periods in environments with low humidity, such as airplane cabins or excessively dry office spaces, can exacerbate the condition.

Age: As individuals age, the natural production of tears tends to decrease. This can lead to a higher prevalence of dry eye in older adults, particularly in women after menopause, due to hormonal changes.

Medications: Certain medications, including antihistamines, decongestants, diuretics, beta-blockers, and antidepressants, can disrupt tear production or increase tear evaporation, leading to dry eye symptoms.

Medical Conditions: Various medical conditions and systemic diseases can contribute to the development of dry eye syndrome. Autoimmune diseases like Sjögren's syndrome, rheumatoid arthritis, and lupus can affect the body's ability to produce tears effectively. Other conditions such as diabetes, thyroid disorders, and vitamin A deficiency can also be associated with dry eye.

Digital Device Usage: The widespread use of computers, smartphones, and other digital devices has led to an increase in cases of digital eye strain and dry eye. Prolonged screen time can reduce blink rate, leading to inadequate tear distribution and increased evaporation.

Contact Lens Wear: Wearing contact lenses can exacerbate dry eye symptoms, as they may disrupt the tear film and cause increased tear evaporation. Individuals who experience dry eye with contact lens wear should seek advice from their eye care professionals on proper lens selection and care.

Meibomian Gland Dysfunction (MGD): Dysfunction of the meibomian glands, responsible for producing the oily component of tears, can lead to evaporative dry eye. When the oils are not adequately released onto the tear film, it becomes unstable, leading to increased tear evaporation.

Eyelid Conditions: Anatomical abnormalities or conditions affecting the eyelids, such as blepharitis (inflammation of the eyelids) or ectropion (outward-turning eyelid), can disrupt the distribution and secretion of tears, contributing to dry eye.

LASIK Surgery: Some individuals may experience temporary dry eye symptoms after undergoing LASIK or other refractive eye surgeries, as the corneal nerves responsible for signaling tear production can be affected during the procedure.

Hormonal Changes: Hormonal fluctuations, particularly in women during pregnancy or menopause, can lead to changes in tear production and composition, resulting in dry eye symptoms.

By understanding these causes and risk factors, individuals can take proactive measures to prevent or manage dry eye syndrome. If experiencing persistent or severe dry eye symptoms, it is essential to consult an eye care professional for a comprehensive evaluation and personalized treatment plan.

Different Types Of Dry Eye Conditions

Dry eye syndrome is not a one-size-fits-all condition, and there are different types of dry eye conditions, each with its unique underlying causes and characteristics. Understanding these distinctions is crucial in tailoring effective treatment plans.
 Below are the primary types of dry eye conditions:

Evaporative Dry Eye:

Evaporative dry eye is the most common type and occurs when the tears evaporate too quickly due to inadequate oil production from the meibomian glands. These glands are located in the eyelids and secrete oils that help form the outermost layer of the tear film, reducing tear evaporation. Dysfunction of the meibomian glands, often referred to as meibomian gland dysfunction (MGD), can lead to an unstable tear film and contribute to dry eye symptoms. People with evaporative dry eye may experience gritty or sandy sensations in their eyes, discomfort, and fluctuating vision.

Aqueous-Deficient Dry Eye:

Aqueous-deficient dry eye, also known as tear-deficient dry eye, is characterized by a lack of adequate tear production from the lacrimal glands, which are responsible for producing the watery component of tears. Reduced tear volume can lead to insufficient lubrication of the ocular surface, resulting in dryness, irritation, and blurred vision. Aqueous-deficient dry eye can be caused by various factors, including certain medical conditions, systemic diseases, or ocular surface inflammation.

Mixed Dry Eye:

Mixed dry eye is a combination of both evaporative and aqueous-deficient dry eye. This type of dry eye occurs when there are issues with both the meibomian glands' oil production and the lacrimal glands' tear production. Individuals with mixed dry eye may experience a variety of symptoms that can be challenging to manage due to the dual factors contributing to the condition.

Non-Sjögren's Dry Eye:
Sjögren's syndrome is an autoimmune disease that primarily affects the salivary and lacrimal glands, leading to dry mouth and dry eyes. However, not all cases of dry eye are related to Sjögren's syndrome. Non-Sjögren's dry eye refers to dry eye conditions that are not associated with this specific autoimmune disorder but share similar symptoms and mechanisms. It can result from various environmental, hormonal, or medical factors, as mentioned earlier.

Seasonal Dry Eye:
Some individuals experience dry eye symptoms that are closely tied to specific seasons, typically exacerbated by environmental factors such as low humidity, increased pollen, and allergens. Seasonal dry eye can be more prominent in certain climates and may require targeted management during specific times of the year.

Understanding the specific type of dry eye is crucial in developing an effective treatment plan. Eye care professionals can perform comprehensive evaluations, including tear film assessments and meibomian gland expression, to determine the primary factors contributing to the dry eye condition. Based on the diagnosis, a tailored approach can be implemented, including lifestyle modifications, artificial tears, eyelid hygiene, anti-inflammatory treatments, or other therapies, to provide relief and improve overall eye health.

Impact Of Dry Eye On Overall Eye Health

Dry eye syndrome can have a significant impact on overall eye health, affecting various aspects of ocular function and comfort. When the eyes lack adequate lubrication and nourishment, a range of complications can arise, leading to potential long-term consequences.

Here are some ways dry eye can impact overall eye health:

Corneal Damage: The cornea, the clear front surface of the eye, relies on a smooth and continuous tear film for optimal vision. In cases of chronic dry eye, the lack of proper lubrication can lead to corneal damage. Abrasions, scratches, and erosion of the corneal epithelium may occur, causing discomfort and vision disturbances.

Vision Disturbances: Dry eye can cause vision fluctuations, particularly when blinking. As the tear film becomes unstable, light refraction can be affected, leading to blurred or hazy vision. Individuals may also experience difficulty focusing, especially during prolonged reading or computer use.

Eye Infections: Tears have a protective function by flushing away debris and potentially harmful microorganisms from the ocular surface. In cases of dry eye, the reduced tear flow and compromised tear quality may result in an increased risk of eye infections, such as conjunctivitis or keratitis.

Eye Fatigue: Prolonged periods of dryness and discomfort can lead to eye fatigue, making it challenging to sustain visual tasks comfortably. Activities like reading, using digital devices, or driving may become more burdensome for individuals with dry eye.

Reduced Tear Production: In some cases, chronic dry eye can lead to a vicious cycle, where the ocular surface inflammation caused by the condition further reduces tear production. This cycle can exacerbate dry eye symptoms and make the condition more challenging to manage.

Impact on Quality of Life: Dry eye can significantly impact a person's quality of life. The discomfort, irritation, and visual disturbances associated with the condition can interfere with daily activities and reduce productivity and overall well-being.

Psychological Effects: Chronic dry eye can lead to emotional distress, frustration, and anxiety, particularly when the symptoms persist despite efforts to alleviate them. Coping with a chronic eye condition can have psychological ramifications, affecting an individual's mental health and self-esteem.

It is essential to address dry eye promptly and adequately to prevent further complications and discomfort. Seeking professional advice from an eye care specialist can help identify the underlying causes of dry eye and tailor a treatment plan to manage the condition effectively. Depending on the type and severity of dry eye, treatments may include artificial tears, lubricating ointments, lifestyle modifications, anti-inflammatory medications, and in some cases, specialized procedures or therapies to address specific contributing factors.

Regular eye examinations and early intervention are essential to maintaining eye health and managing dry eye syndrome effectively. By addressing the impact of dry eye on overall eye health, individuals can improve their comfort, vision, and quality of life.

CHAPTER 2: SIGNS AND SYMPTOMS

In this chapter, we will explore the various signs and symptoms associated with dry eye, providing insights into recognizing and understanding this common ocular condition. Differentiating dry eye from other eye conditions is crucial in ensuring proper diagnosis and appropriate management.

Recognizing The Signs Of Dry Eye

Recognizing the signs of dry eye is essential in identifying the condition early and seeking appropriate management. Dry eye syndrome can present with various ocular manifestations, and being aware of these signs can help individuals seek timely evaluation from an eye care professional.

Here are some key signs to watch for:

Eye Redness: One of the prominent signs of dry eye is redness in the eyes. The blood vessels on the ocular surface may become more visible due to inflammation and irritation caused by insufficient tear film.

Fluctuating Vision: Dry eye can lead to intermittent changes in vision clarity. Vision may vary throughout the day, particularly during activities that demand prolonged visual focus, such as reading, using digital devices, or driving.

Sensation of Dryness: The hallmark symptom of dry eye is a persistent sensation of dryness in the eyes. This discomfort may feel like a scratchy, gritty, or sandy feeling, as if there is something in the eye.

Excessive Tearing: Surprisingly, dry eye can lead to reflex tearing, where the eyes produce an overflow of tears as a compensatory response to the lack of proper lubrication.

Light Sensitivity: Individuals with dry eye may experience increased sensitivity to light, known as photophobia. Bright lights or sunlight can exacerbate the discomfort and make it difficult to keep the eyes open comfortably.

Discomfort During Visual Tasks: Dry eye symptoms may worsen during visually demanding tasks, such as reading or using digital screens for extended periods.

Foreign Body Sensation: Some people with dry eye may experience a feeling of a foreign body or something stuck in their eye, leading to frequent blinking or rubbing.

Tired Eyes: Dry eye can cause eye fatigue and a sense of heaviness or tiredness in the eyes, even after minimal visual tasks.

Watery Eyes: Paradoxically, dry eye can lead to increased reflex tearing, which may cause eyes to water excessively without providing relief from the underlying dryness.

If you experience one or more of these signs consistently or notice a decline in your overall eye comfort, it is essential to seek advice from an eye care professional. An eye examination can help diagnose dry eye and determine the appropriate course of action to manage and alleviate your symptoms effectively. Early detection and treatment can prevent potential complications and improve your overall eye health and quality of life.

Common Symptoms And Their Severity

Common symptoms of dry eye syndrome can vary in severity among individuals. The intensity of symptoms can fluctuate based on factors such as environmental conditions, lifestyle habits, and overall eye health.
 Here are the most prevalent symptoms and their potential severity:

Mild Dryness: Some individuals may experience occasional mild dryness in the eyes, which may be more noticeable during specific activities or in certain environments. The discomfort may be tolerable and may not significantly impact daily activities.

Moderate Discomfort: Moderate dry eye symptoms can include a persistent sensation of dryness, grittiness, or a foreign body sensation in the eyes. The discomfort may be more pronounced during visual tasks like reading or using digital devices for extended periods. Artificial tear use or eye drops may provide temporary relief.

Burning and Stinging: For some individuals, dry eye can cause a burning or stinging sensation in the eyes. The discomfort may become more bothersome, particularly in dry or windy environments or when exposed to air conditioning or heating systems.

Intermittent Blurred Vision: Dry eye can lead to intermittent blurred vision, especially during activities that demand sustained visual focus. The blurriness may improve temporarily with blinking or the use of artificial tears.

Excessive Tearing: In response to dryness and irritation, the eyes may produce excessive reflex tears, leading to watery eyes. Paradoxically, this excess tearing does not provide sufficient lubrication, and the eyes may still feel dry and uncomfortable.

Severe Dryness and Irritation: In severe cases of dry eye, the discomfort can become intense and constant, significantly impacting daily life and visual tasks. The eyes may feel extremely dry and irritated, leading to increased sensitivity to light and difficulty keeping the eyes open comfortably.

Corneal Damage: If left untreated, chronic dry eye can lead to corneal damage, with symptoms such as increased corneal staining, corneal erosions, or recurrent eye infections. Severe corneal damage may cause significant vision disturbances and require specialized treatment.

It is essential to recognize and monitor the severity of dry eye symptoms to determine the appropriate management and seek timely professional advice. Over-the-counter artificial tears can provide relief for mild to moderate symptoms. However, for more severe or persistent symptoms, it is advisable to consult an eye care professional for a comprehensive evaluation and personalized treatment plan.

Proactive management of dry eye can help improve comfort, preserve visual function, and prevent potential complications that may arise from untreated or inadequately managed dry eye syndrome. Regular follow-up with an eye care professional is crucial to monitor the condition and adjust treatment strategies as needed to maintain overall eye health and well-being.

How To Distinguish Dry Eye From Other Eye Conditions

Distinguishing dry eye from other eye conditions is essential in ensuring accurate diagnosis and appropriate management. Several eye conditions can share similar symptoms, but each requires specific treatment approaches. Here are some key considerations and methods to distinguish dry eye from other eye conditions:

Comprehensive Eye Examination: A thorough eye examination by an eye care professional is crucial in identifying the underlying cause of your symptoms. During the examination, the eye care professional will assess the health of your eyes, including the tear film, cornea, conjunctiva, and eyelids.

Tear Film Assessment: An evaluation of the tear film quality and quantity can provide valuable insights. Tear breakup time (TBUT) measures the stability of the tear film, and a shorter TBUT may indicate dry eye. Tear production can be measured using Schirmer's test, which involves placing a strip of filter paper on the lower eyelid to measure tear volume.

Meibomian Gland Evaluation: Dysfunction of the meibomian glands is common in dry eye. An examination of the eyelids and meibomian gland expression can help identify potential issues related to meibomian gland dysfunction (MGD).

Differentiation from Allergic Conjunctivitis: Allergic conjunctivitis can cause redness, itching, and excessive tearing, which may be similar to dry eye symptoms. However, in allergic conjunctivitis, symptoms are typically seasonal and related to allergen exposure. Allergy testing or a detailed medical history can aid in distinguishing the two conditions.

Evaluation for Conjunctivitis and Infections: Infectious conjunctivitis (pink eye) and other eye infections may also present with redness, tearing, and discomfort. The presence of discharge or crusting, along with a recent history of exposure to infections, may point towards an infectious cause rather than dry eye.

Assessment for Other Ocular Conditions: Conditions such as blepharitis, corneal abrasions, and conjunctival abnormalities can mimic some dry eye symptoms. Differentiating dry eye from these conditions requires a comprehensive eye examination and specific diagnostic tests.

Response to Treatment: The response to initial treatment can provide valuable information. If the symptoms improve with artificial tears and other dry eye management strategies, it suggests dry eye as the primary condition. On the other hand, if there is no improvement or worsening of symptoms, reevaluation for other possible eye conditions may be necessary.

Underlying Medical Conditions: Certain systemic conditions, such as Sjögren's syndrome or autoimmune disorders, can cause dry eye symptoms. A detailed medical history and additional testing may be needed to identify such conditions.

Seeking professional advice from an eye care specialist is vital for accurate diagnosis and appropriate management. An experienced eye care professional can perform the necessary tests and examinations to distinguish dry eye from other eye conditions and create a personalized treatment plan tailored to your specific needs. Early diagnosis and targeted management can help alleviate symptoms, improve overall eye health, and enhance your quality of life.

CHAPTER 3: THE IMPORTANCE OF HOLISTIC APPROACH TO DRY EYE

In this chapter, we will delve into the significance of adopting a holistic approach in managing dry eye. Understanding the interconnections between various aspects of health and lifestyle can provide valuable insights into improving the overall well-being of individuals experiencing dry eye symptoms. We will explore the relevance of holistic health, the mind-body connection, and the influence of lifestyle, diet, and environment on dry eye.

Exploring Holistic Health And Its Relevance To Dry Eye

Exploring holistic health and its relevance to dry eye involves recognizing that the condition is influenced by interconnected factors beyond the ocular surface. Holistic health focuses on the integration of physical, mental, emotional, and environmental well-being to achieve overall wellness. By applying this approach to dry eye management, individuals can gain valuable insights into the various aspects of their lives that may impact the condition.

Here are the key aspects of exploring holistic health in relation to dry eye:

Systemic Health and Dry Eye:
Holistic health acknowledges that the health of the entire body can influence specific conditions, including dry eye. Underlying systemic health issues, such as autoimmune disorders, diabetes, and hormonal imbalances, can affect tear production and ocular surface health. Addressing these systemic conditions can play a crucial role in managing dry eye effectively.

Stress and Emotional Well-being:
Stress and emotional factors can impact the ocular surface and tear film, leading to or exacerbating dry eye symptoms. The mind-body connection illustrates how emotional well-being can affect physical health. High levels of stress can reduce tear production and increase eye discomfort. Incorporating stress management techniques, such as mindfulness, meditation, or yoga, can help reduce stress and positively influence dry eye symptoms.

Nutrition and Lifestyle Choices:
Diet and lifestyle play essential roles in overall health, including eye health. A balanced diet rich in omega-3 fatty

acids, antioxidants, and hydration can support tear production and maintain a healthy ocular surface. Conversely, poor dietary choices, smoking, and excessive alcohol consumption can contribute to dry eye symptoms. Exploring dietary and lifestyle modifications can aid in managing dry eye holistically.

Environmental Factors:

Environmental conditions can impact dry eye. Prolonged exposure to air conditioning, heating, dry climates, or excessive digital device usage can lead to increased tear evaporation and dry eye symptoms. Understanding and adjusting environmental factors can help alleviate dry eye discomfort.

Sleep Quality:

Quality sleep is crucial for overall health, including eye health. Sleep patterns and habits can influence dry eye symptoms, as insufficient sleep can lead to reduced tear production and increased ocular irritation. Focusing on improving sleep hygiene and obtaining adequate rest can positively affect dry eye management.

Mindfulness and Self-Care:

Practicing mindfulness and self-care can reduce stress and promote emotional well-being. Engaging in activities that bring joy and relaxation can positively impact dry eye symptoms by reducing stress-related exacerbations.

Embracing a holistic approach to dry eye management involves considering the interplay between physical health, emotional well-being, lifestyle, and the environment. By exploring these interconnected factors, individuals can develop personalized strategies to address dry eye effectively. Integrating stress reduction techniques, dietary adjustments, and lifestyle modifications with traditional dry eye treatments can lead to improved overall eye comfort and quality of life. A comprehensive approach to dry eye management empowers individuals to take a proactive role in supporting their eye health and well-being.

Understanding The Mind-body Connection

Understanding the mind-body connection is a fundamental aspect of holistic health and wellness. It acknowledges the interrelationship between our mental and emotional states and their impact on our physical well-being. This connection highlights how thoughts, emotions, and behaviors can influence various physiological processes in the body, including those related to health and disease. Here are key points to comprehend the mind-body connection:

Thoughts and Emotions Influence Physiology:

Our thoughts and emotions can trigger physical responses in the body. For example, feelings of stress, anxiety, or fear can activate the body's "fight or flight" response, leading to increased heart rate, elevated blood pressure, and a release of stress hormones like cortisol. Conversely, positive emotions such as happiness, joy, and relaxation can trigger the body's relaxation response, promoting feelings of calmness and well-being.

Impact on Immune Function:

The mind-body connection can influence the immune system. Chronic stress and negative emotions can suppress immune function, making individuals more susceptible to infections and illnesses. On the other hand, positive emotions and a healthy mental state can strengthen the immune system, supporting overall health and resilience.

Effects on Chronic Conditions:

The mind-body connection plays a significant role in chronic conditions and their management. For instance, stress and negative emotions can exacerbate symptoms of conditions like asthma, irritable bowel syndrome (IBS), and chronic pain. Managing stress and adopting positive coping strategies can improve the management of these conditions.

Stress and Inflammation:
Chronic stress can lead to increased inflammation in the body. Inflammation is a natural immune response, but persistent inflammation can contribute to the development of various health conditions, including cardiovascular disease, diabetes, and autoimmune disorders.

Mindfulness and Relaxation Techniques:
Practices like mindfulness meditation, deep breathing, and progressive muscle relaxation are examples of techniques that leverage the mind-body connection to reduce stress and promote relaxation. These practices can positively impact overall health, including eye health, by reducing stress-related exacerbations of conditions like dry eye.

Placebo and Nocebo Effects:
The mind-body connection also influences the placebo and nocebo effects. The placebo effect refers to improvements in

symptoms or health conditions observed when individuals believe they are receiving treatment, even if the treatment is inactive. Conversely, the nocebo effect occurs when negative outcomes or symptoms are experienced due to negative expectations or beliefs.

Understanding the mind-body connection empowers individuals to take an active role in their health and well-being. By cultivating positive emotions, managing stress, and engaging in relaxation practices, individuals can positively impact their physical health, including conditions like dry eye. Integrating mindfulness and self-care practices into dry eye management can enhance the effectiveness of treatment strategies and improve overall eye comfort and quality of life.

How Lifestyle, Diet, And Environment Influence Dry Eye

Lifestyle, diet, and environment play significant roles in influencing dry eye symptoms and overall eye health. These factors can impact tear production, tear quality, and the stability of the tear film, all of which are crucial for maintaining a healthy ocular surface. Understanding how lifestyle, diet, and environment influence dry eye can help individuals make informed choices to manage and alleviate their symptoms effectively.

Lifestyle Factors:

1. Digital Device Usage: Prolonged use of computers, smartphones, and other digital devices can lead to reduced blink rate and incomplete blinking, which can contribute to dry eye symptoms. The reduced blinking leads to inadequate tear distribution across the ocular surface, resulting in dryness and discomfort.

2. Smoking: Smoking has been linked to an increased risk of developing dry eye syndrome. The chemicals in tobacco smoke can irritate the eyes and disrupt the tear film, leading to dryness and ocular discomfort.

3. Indoor Environments: Spending extended periods in environments with air conditioning or heating systems can reduce indoor humidity, leading to dry air that can accelerate tear evaporation and worsen dry eye symptoms.

4. Outdoor Environments: Exposure to windy and dry climates can also contribute to dry eye symptoms as the wind can increase tear evaporation.

Diet and Nutrition:

1. Omega-3 Fatty Acids: Omega-3 fatty acids, found in fatty fish (e.g., salmon, tuna, sardines) and certain nuts and seeds, are essential for maintaining a healthy tear film and reducing inflammation in the eyes. A diet rich in omega-3s can support tear production and alleviate dry eye symptoms.

2. Hydration: Staying well-hydrated is essential for overall health and can help maintain an adequate tear film. Drinking sufficient water throughout the day can promote proper tear lubrication and ocular comfort.

3. Antioxidants: Consuming a diet rich in antioxidants from fruits and vegetables can help protect the eyes from oxidative stress and inflammation.

Environmental Factors:

1. Humidity: Dry and low-humidity environments can promote increased tear evaporation, exacerbating dry eye symptoms. In such conditions, using a humidifier can help maintain indoor humidity levels and reduce ocular discomfort.

2. Allergens: Allergens like pollen, dust, and pet dander can trigger dry eye symptoms in individuals with allergic reactions. Minimizing exposure to allergens and using allergy eye drops can help manage dry eye related to allergies.

Being mindful of these lifestyle, diet, and environmental factors can help individuals take proactive steps to manage dry eye. Implementing lifestyle modifications, maintaining a balanced diet, and making adjustments to the indoor environment can complement traditional dry eye treatments, providing relief and improving overall eye comfort. Consulting an eye care professional for personalized advice on managing dry eye based on individual needs and circumstances is recommended.

CHAPTER 4: NOURISHING YOUR EYES: NUTRITION FOR DRY EYE RELIEF

In this chapter, we will explore the essential nutrients for maintaining eye health, focusing on their relevance in alleviating dry eye symptoms. Understanding the importance of a well-balanced diet and eye-friendly foods can provide valuable insights into nourishing your eyes for optimal dry eye relief. We will discuss the nutrients vital for eye health, eye-friendly foods, and supplements, along with tips for creating a dry eye-friendly diet plan.

Nutrients Essential For Eye Health

Several nutrients are essential for maintaining eye health and supporting optimal vision. These nutrients play critical roles in protecting the eyes from oxidative damage, maintaining the health of the ocular structures, and promoting overall visual function.

Here are some of the key nutrients that are beneficial for eye health:

Vitamin A: Vitamin A is essential for the health of the retina, the light-sensitive tissue at the back of the eye that plays a crucial role in vision. It helps maintain the surface of the eye (cornea) and supports low-light vision. Foods rich in vitamin A include carrots, sweet potatoes, spinach, kale, and other leafy green vegetables.

Vitamin C: As a powerful antioxidant, vitamin C helps protect the eyes from oxidative stress and supports the health of blood vessels in the eye. It is abundant in citrus fruits (oranges, grapefruits), strawberries, bell peppers, broccoli, and kiwi.

Vitamin E: Vitamin E is another potent antioxidant that helps protect cells in the eyes from damage caused by free radicals. It supports eye health by promoting healthy cell membranes. Foods rich in vitamin E include almonds, sunflower seeds, vegetable oils (such as sunflower oil), and leafy greens.

Omega-3 Fatty Acids: Omega-3s are essential for maintaining a healthy tear film, reducing inflammation in the eyes, and supporting the overall health of the ocular surface. These fatty acids are particularly beneficial for individuals experiencing dry eye symptoms. Fatty fish like salmon, mackerel, and trout are excellent sources of omega-3s. Plant-based sources include chia seeds, flaxseeds, and walnuts.

Zinc: Zinc is essential for transporting vitamin A from the liver to the retina, where it is required for optimal visual function. Zinc also plays a role in the metabolism of antioxidants in the eye. Foods rich in zinc include meat (beef, lamb, poultry), shellfish (oysters, crab, shrimp), pumpkin seeds, and legumes (chickpeas, lentils).

Lutein and Zeaxanthin: These two antioxidants are carotenoids that accumulate in the retina, where they help protect against harmful high-energy light waves (blue light) and reduce the risk of age-related macular degeneration (AMD). Leafy greens, such as spinach, kale, and collard greens, are excellent sources of lutein and zeaxanthin.

Copper: Copper is involved in the formation of melanin, a pigment found in the eyes that helps protect against UV light. It also plays a role in the maintenance of connective tissues in the eye. Copper is present in a variety of foods, including shellfish, nuts, seeds, and whole grains.

Including a wide variety of nutrient-rich foods in your diet can help ensure you obtain the essential nutrients needed for maintaining eye health. Additionally, if you have specific eye health concerns or dietary restrictions, consulting with an eye care professional or a registered dietitian can provide personalized guidance on how to optimize your diet for optimal eye health.

Eye-friendly Foods And Supplements

Eye-friendly foods and supplements are those that contain essential nutrients beneficial for maintaining good eye health and supporting optimal vision. Including these foods in your diet or considering appropriate supplements can provide the necessary vitamins, minerals, and antioxidants to promote eye wellness. Here are some eye-friendly foods and supplements to consider:

Eye-Friendly Foods:

1. Fatty Fish: Fatty fish like salmon, mackerel, trout, and sardines are rich sources of omega-3 fatty acids, specifically DHA (docosahexaenoic acid) and EPA (eicosapentaenoic acid). These omega-3s support the health of the retina, reduce inflammation in the eyes, and contribute to a healthy tear film. Regular consumption of fatty fish can be beneficial for individuals with dry eyes or those looking to support overall eye health.

2. Leafy Greens: Spinach, kale, collard greens, and other leafy green vegetables are excellent sources of lutein and zeaxanthin, two powerful antioxidants that accumulate in the retina. Lutein and zeaxanthin help protect the eyes from harmful high-energy light waves (blue light) and may reduce the risk of age-related macular degeneration (AMD). Including these leafy greens in your diet can be particularly beneficial for maintaining macular health.

3. Citrus Fruits and Berries: Citrus fruits (oranges, grapefruits) and berries (strawberries, blueberries, blackberries) are rich in vitamin C, a potent antioxidant that helps protect the eyes from oxidative stress and supports healthy blood vessels. These fruits are easy to incorporate into your diet and can provide a tasty and nutritious addition to meals and snacks.

4. Nuts and Seeds: Almonds, walnuts, chia seeds, and flaxseeds are good sources of vitamin E and omega-3 fatty acids. Vitamin E is an antioxidant that helps protect cells in the eyes from damage caused by free radicals. Including a variety of nuts and seeds in your diet can provide essential nutrients for eye health.

Eye-Friendly Supplements:

1. Omega-3 Supplements: For individuals who have difficulty obtaining sufficient omega-3s from their diet, omega-3 supplements can be a convenient option. Fish oil supplements or vegetarian alternatives derived from algae can provide DHA and EPA to support eye health and alleviate dry eye symptoms.

2. Lutein and Zeaxanthin Supplements: If it is challenging to consume enough leafy greens rich in lutein and zeaxanthin, supplements containing these carotenoids can be considered to support macular health and protect against AMD.

3. Vitamin C and E Supplements: Vitamin C and E supplements can be beneficial for individuals who have specific dietary restrictions or require additional antioxidant support for their eyes.

When considering supplements, it is essential to consult with an eye care professional or a registered dietitian to ensure the appropriate dosage and to determine if supplementation is necessary based on individual needs and health conditions. Supplements should not replace a well-balanced diet but can complement it to support overall eye health and well-being.

Creating A Dry Eye-friendly Diet Plan

Creating a dry eye-friendly diet plan involves incorporating nutrient-rich foods that support eye health and alleviate dry eye symptoms. By focusing on specific nutrients and antioxidants, individuals can optimize their diet to nourish their eyes and maintain a healthy tear film. Here are key steps to create a dry eye-friendly diet plan:

Prioritize Omega-3 Fatty Acids: Omega-3s are crucial for reducing inflammation and supporting tear production. Include fatty fish like salmon, mackerel, and trout in your diet at least twice a week. For those with dietary restrictions or preferences, consider plant-based sources of omega-3s like chia seeds, flaxseeds, and walnuts.

Load Up on Leafy Greens: Leafy green vegetables like spinach, kale, and collard greens are rich in lutein and zeaxanthin, which protect against harmful blue light and

45

support macular health. Incorporate these greens into salads, smoothies, or sautés regularly.

Include Colorful Fruits and Vegetables: Vibrant fruits and vegetables, such as carrots, sweet potatoes, bell peppers, berries, and citrus fruits, provide essential vitamins (A and C) and antioxidants that promote eye health. Aim for a rainbow of colors in your meals to ensure a diverse nutrient intake.

Add Nuts and Seeds: Almonds, walnuts, chia seeds, and flaxseeds are excellent sources of vitamin E and omega-3s. Sprinkle nuts and seeds on salads, yogurt, or oatmeal to enhance nutritional value.

Choose Healthy Fats: Opt for heart-healthy fats like olive oil, avocados, and olives. These fats support overall health and can help absorb fat-soluble vitamins essential for eye health.

Hydration is Key: Stay well-hydrated throughout the day by drinking plenty of water. Proper hydration supports tear lubrication and reduces the risk of dry eye discomfort.

Limit Processed and Sugary Foods: Minimize the intake of processed and sugary foods, as they may contribute to inflammation and do not provide adequate nutrition for eye health. Instead, opt for whole foods that offer a wide range of nutrients.

Consider Supplements: If it is challenging to obtain sufficient nutrients from your diet, consult with an eye care professional or a registered dietitian about appropriate supplements. Omega-3 supplements, vitamin C, vitamin E, and lutein/zeaxanthin supplements can complement your diet to support eye health.

Manage Portion Sizes: Be mindful of portion sizes to maintain a balanced diet and prevent overeating, which can lead to weight gain and potential metabolic issues that may affect eye health.

Practice Consistency: Establishing healthy eating habits and maintaining a balanced diet is a gradual process. Be consistent in incorporating eye-friendly foods into your meals and strive for long-term dietary changes that promote eye health.

Creating a dry eye-friendly diet plan is a proactive approach to managing dry eye symptoms and supporting overall eye health. Remember that a healthy diet is just one component of a comprehensive dry eye management plan. For personalized guidance, consult with an eye care professional or a registered dietitian who can tailor recommendations based on your individual needs and health status.

CHAPTER 5: HYDRATION AND EYE HEALTH

In this chapter, we will explore the crucial role of proper hydration in preventing dry eye and supporting overall eye health. Understanding the relationship between water intake and eye moisture can help individuals maintain optimal hydration for their eyes. We will also provide practical tips for staying hydrated throughout the day to promote eye health and prevent dry eye symptoms.

The Role Of Proper Hydration In Preventing Dry Eye

Proper hydration plays a vital role in preventing dry eye and maintaining overall eye health. The eyes rely on a well-hydrated tear film to keep the ocular surface lubricated, nourished, and protected. When the body is adequately hydrated, the tear film remains stable, and the eyes are less likely to experience dryness, discomfort, and irritation. Here's an in-depth look at the role of proper hydration in preventing dry eye:

Tear Film Maintenance: The tear film is a complex structure that covers the surface of the eye. It consists of three layers: the lipid (oil) layer, the aqueous (water) layer, and the mucin (mucus) layer. Each layer plays a specific role in tear stability and function. Adequate hydration helps maintain the proper balance of these layers, ensuring that the tear film covers the ocular surface effectively.

Tear Production: Proper hydration is essential for tear production. Tears are composed mostly of water, and when the body is dehydrated, tear production may decrease, leading to dry eye symptoms. Ensuring sufficient water intake supports the body's ability to produce an adequate volume of tears to keep the eyes moist and comfortable.

Ocular Surface Protection: Tears act as a protective barrier for the eyes, preventing foreign particles, irritants, and pathogens from sticking to the ocular surface. A well-hydrated tear film enhances this protective function, reducing the risk of eye infections and discomfort.

Blinking and Tear Distribution: Dehydration can affect the blink rate and the efficiency of blinking. Inadequate blinking can lead to an uneven distribution of tears across the ocular surface, contributing to dry spots and discomfort.

Staying well-hydrated encourages regular blinking, which helps distribute tears evenly, promoting eye moisture.

Environmental Factors: Dry and low-humidity environments can increase tear evaporation, leading to dry eye symptoms. Proper hydration can help counteract the effects of dry environments by maintaining the tear film's moisture and reducing evaporation.

Prevention of Ocular Irritation: Dry eye can cause eye redness, irritation, and a foreign body sensation. Ensuring proper hydration reduces the likelihood of these discomforts and allows individuals to enjoy more comfortable and healthier eyes.

To maintain proper hydration for preventing dry eye, it is essential to drink an adequate amount of water throughout the day. Individual hydration needs may vary based on factors such as age, activity level, and climate. Listening to the body's thirst signals and paying attention to urine color can help gauge hydration status. Additionally, avoiding excessive consumption of dehydrating beverages like caffeine and alcohol and including water-rich fruits and vegetables in the diet can further support eye hydration.

For individuals experiencing persistent or severe dry eye symptoms, consulting with an eye care professional is recommended. Proper hydration, along with other dry eye management strategies, can significantly improve eye comfort and contribute to better overall eye health.

Water Intake And Its Impact On Eye Moisture

Water intake has a direct impact on eye moisture and the health of the tear film. The tear film is a thin layer of fluid that covers the surface of the eyes, providing essential lubrication and nourishment to maintain optimal eye comfort and function. Adequate water intake is crucial for maintaining the right balance of tears, preventing dry eye, and supporting overall eye health. Here's how water intake impacts eye moisture:

Tear Production: Tears are mostly composed of water, along with other essential components like proteins, lipids, and mucins. When the body is well-hydrated, it can produce a sufficient volume of tears to keep the eyes moist and comfortable. Insufficient water intake can lead to reduced tear production, resulting in dry eye symptoms such as itching, burning, and a gritty sensation.

Tear Stability: The tear film consists of three layers: the lipid (oil) layer, the aqueous (water) layer, and the mucin (mucus) layer. Each layer plays a critical role in tear stability and function. Adequate water intake helps maintain the necessary water content in tears, contributing to the stability of the tear film. A stable tear film ensures that the eyes stay moist and protected from external irritants.

Tear Evaporation: Tears can evaporate from the ocular surface, especially in dry or low-humidity environments. Dehydration can exacerbate this evaporation process, leading to a rapid decrease in tear volume and an increase in dry eye symptoms. By staying well-hydrated, individuals can minimize tear evaporation and retain the moisture needed to maintain comfortable eyes.

Blinking Efficiency: Proper hydration supports the efficiency of blinking, which is essential for distributing tears evenly across the ocular surface. Regular blinking helps flush out debris and maintains the tear film's integrity. Inadequate hydration can affect blinking patterns, leading to uneven tear distribution and potential dry spots on the eyes.

Eye Comfort and Irritation: When the eyes are well-hydrated, individuals are less likely to experience eye discomfort, redness, and irritation. Dry eyes can lead to feelings of grittiness, burning, or sensitivity to light. Sufficient water intake can help alleviate these symptoms and promote more comfortable and healthier eyes.

To ensure adequate water intake and maintain eye moisture, individuals should aim to drink water regularly throughout the day, even if they do not feel thirsty. Setting reminders or using water bottles as visual cues can be helpful in encouraging consistent hydration. Monitoring urine color is another way to gauge hydration status, as pale yellow urine indicates proper hydration. Additionally, limiting the consumption of dehydrating beverages like caffeine and alcohol can help support optimal eye moisture.

For individuals experiencing chronic or severe dry eye symptoms, seeking guidance from an eye care professional is essential. Proper water intake, combined with other dry eye management strategies, can significantly improve eye comfort and contribute to better eye health.

Tips For Maintaining Eye Hydration Throughout The Day

Maintaining eye hydration throughout the day is essential for preventing dry eye and promoting overall eye health. By incorporating simple habits and strategies, individuals can ensure that their eyes stay moist and comfortable. Here are some practical tips for maintaining eye hydration throughout the day:

Drink Plenty of Water: The most straightforward and effective way to maintain eye hydration is to drink plenty of water throughout the day. Aim to consume at least eight glasses (about 64 ounces) of water daily. Keeping a water bottle with you can serve as a reminder to stay hydrated.

Set Hydration Reminders: In today's busy world, it can be easy to forget to drink water. Use alarms or mobile apps to set hydration reminders at regular intervals, prompting you to take a sip of water.

Listen to Your Thirst: Pay attention to your body's thirst signals and drink water when you feel thirsty. Thirst is a natural indicator that your body needs hydration.

Monitor Urine Color: Urine color can be an indicator of hydration status. Aim for pale yellow urine, which suggests proper hydration. Dark yellow urine may indicate dehydration.

Hydrate During Meals: Drink water during meals to complement the hydration you get from food. This can also help with digestion and nutrient absorption.

Include Hydrating Foods: Consume foods with high water content, such as watermelon, cucumber, oranges, grapes, and celery. These fruits and vegetables provide additional hydration throughout the day.

Limit Dehydrating Beverages: Minimize the consumption of dehydrating beverages like caffeine and alcohol. These drinks can contribute to fluid loss and dryness. If you consume caffeinated or alcoholic beverages, balance them with water intake.

Use a Humidifier: If you spend significant time indoors, especially in environments with air conditioning or heating, consider using a humidifier. Humidifiers add moisture to the air, reducing the risk of tear evaporation in dry indoor settings.

Blink Regularly: Blinking is essential for distributing tears across the ocular surface. During prolonged screen use or focused activities, remember to blink regularly to prevent dry spots on the eyes.

Take Breaks from Screens: Prolonged screen use can lead to reduced blinking and increased dry eye symptoms. Follow the 20-20-20 rule: Every 20 minutes, take a 20-second break, and look at something 20 feet away. This can help reduce eye strain and promote eye moisture.

Avoid Overexposure to Dry Air: When outdoors in dry or windy conditions, consider wearing sunglasses or protective eyewear to shield your eyes from wind and dust, which can accelerate tear evaporation.

Protect Your Eyes from UV Rays: Wear sunglasses that offer UV protection to shield your eyes from harmful UV rays. UV exposure can contribute to eye dryness and discomfort.

By incorporating these tips into your daily routine, you can maintain optimal eye hydration, reduce the risk of dry eye symptoms, and support overall eye health. If you experience persistent or severe dry eye symptoms, consider consulting with an eye care professional for personalized guidance and treatment.

CHAPTER 6: LIFESTYLE ADJUSTMENTS FOR DRY EYE RELIEF

In this chapter, we will explore lifestyle adjustments that can provide relief from dry eye symptoms. By implementing eye hygiene practices, managing screen time, and adopting stress reduction techniques, individuals can proactively alleviate dry eye discomfort and improve overall eye health.

Eye Hygiene Practices To Alleviate Symptoms

Eye hygiene practices are essential for alleviating dry eye symptoms and maintaining good eye health. These practices help keep the eyes clean, reduce the risk of infection, and promote a stable tear film. By incorporating proper eye hygiene into your daily routine, you can effectively manage dry eye discomfort and prevent potential eye-related issues. Here are some eye hygiene practices to consider:

Wash Hands Thoroughly: Before touching your eyes or applying any eye drops, make sure to wash your hands thoroughly with soap and water. Clean hands help prevent the transfer of germs and dirt to the eyes, reducing the risk of eye infections.

Gently Clean Eyelids: Use a mild, tear-free cleanser or baby shampoo to clean your eyelids daily. Gently apply the cleanser to closed eyelids and use a cotton pad or clean cloth to remove debris and excess oil. This practice helps prevent the buildup of bacteria and reduces the risk of eyelid inflammation (blepharitis).

Use Preservative-Free Eye Drops: If you experience dry eye symptoms, consider using preservative-free artificial tears or lubricating eye drops. These drops provide instant relief by adding moisture to the eyes without causing irritation from preservatives.

Apply Warm Compresses: Using a warm compress can help soothe dry eyes and improve tear film quality. Place a clean, warm, damp cloth over closed eyes for a few minutes, allowing the warmth to facilitate oil gland secretion along the eyelids.

Gentle Lid Massages: Massaging the eyelids can help stimulate the oil glands, improving the quality of the tear film. With clean hands, gently massage your closed eyelids in a circular motion for about 30 seconds.

Avoid Touching or Rubbing Eyes: Refrain from touching or rubbing your eyes, as this can transfer dirt, irritants, and bacteria, potentially worsening dry eye symptoms.

Remove Eye Makeup Properly: When removing eye makeup, use a gentle makeup remover specifically designed for the eyes. Be careful not to tug or pull on the eyelids.

Keep Contact Lenses Clean: If you wear contact lenses, follow proper hygiene practices for their cleaning and storage. Use recommended contact lens solutions and avoid wearing lenses beyond their prescribed duration.

Maintain a Clean Environment: Keep your living and working environments clean and dust-free. Regularly dust and vacuum to reduce the presence of allergens and irritants that may affect the eyes.

Follow Eye Care Professional's Recommendations: If you have specific eye conditions or concerns, follow the advice and recommendations of your eye care professional for proper eye hygiene and management of your eye health.

Remember that every individual's eye health needs are unique. If you experience persistent or severe dry eye symptoms, or if you have any concerns about your eye hygiene practices, consult an eye care professional for personalized guidance and recommendations tailored to your specific situation. Practicing good eye hygiene, along with other dry eye management strategies, can significantly improve eye comfort and contribute to better overall eye health.

Screen Time Management And Its Impact On Dry Eye

Screen time management is crucial for maintaining eye health, especially concerning dry eye symptoms. Prolonged use of digital screens, such as computers, smartphones, tablets, and other electronic devices, can contribute to dry eye discomfort and eye strain. Understanding the impact of screen time on dry eye and adopting appropriate management strategies can help alleviate symptoms and promote overall eye comfort. Here's how screen time affects dry eyes and some tips for effective management:

Impact of Screen Time on Dry Eye:

1. Reduced Blinking: When using digital screens, individuals tend to blink less frequently compared to other activities. Blinking is essential for distributing tears across the ocular surface, ensuring proper eye lubrication. Reduced blinking can lead to evaporative dry eye, where tears evaporate too quickly from the eyes, causing dryness and discomfort.

2. Increased Tear Evaporation: Screens emit blue light, which can contribute to increased tear evaporation and dryness. The proximity of screens to the eyes also intensifies visual demands, leading to eye strain and dry eye symptoms.

3. Decreased Tear Production: Studies suggest that prolonged screen use may reduce tear production. This can further exacerbate dry eye symptoms, leading to redness, irritation, and a gritty sensation.

4. Digital Eye Strain: Extended screen time can cause digital eye strain or computer vision syndrome. Symptoms include eye fatigue, headaches, and blurred vision, which can accompany or contribute to dry eye discomfort.

Tips for Effective Screen Time Management to Alleviate Dry Eye:

1. Follow the 20-20-20 Rule: Take a 20-second break every 20 minutes and focus on something at least 20 feet away. This practice helps reduce eye strain and allows the eyes to rest.

2. Adjust Screen Settings: Ensure that the brightness and contrast levels of your screens are set at comfortable levels. Avoid excessive screen brightness, as it can lead to increased eye strain.

3. Maintain Proper Screen Distance: Position screens at eye level and at an arm's length away. This reduces the need to squint and minimizes eye strain.

4. Use Artificial Tears: Consider using preservative-free artificial tears or lubricating eye drops to keep the eyes moist during prolonged screen time.

5. Reduce Glare: Position screens away from direct sources of light to minimize glare. Anti-glare screens or computer glasses can also help reduce glare and eye strain.

6. Take Regular Breaks: Incorporate breaks in your screen time to give your eyes a rest. Use these breaks to blink regularly, look at something in the distance, or perform eye exercises.

7. Limit Evening Screen Time: Reduce screen time, especially in the evening, to help prevent disrupted sleep patterns, as inadequate sleep can contribute to dry eye symptoms.

8. Maintain Good Posture: Sit in an ergonomically correct position to avoid strain on your neck and shoulders, which can contribute to eye discomfort.

By adopting these screen time management strategies, individuals can reduce the impact of digital devices on dry eyes and promote better eye comfort. Combining these practices with other dry eye management techniques, such as proper eye hygiene and maintaining adequate hydration, can significantly improve overall eye health and well-being. If dry eye symptoms persist or worsen despite these efforts, it is essential to consult with an eye care professional for a comprehensive evaluation and personalized treatment plan.

Techniques For Stress Reduction And Relaxation

Techniques for stress reduction and relaxation are valuable tools for promoting overall well-being, including eye health. High levels of stress can contribute to various health issues, including exacerbating dry eye symptoms and causing eye strain. By incorporating stress reduction techniques into your daily routine, you can alleviate stress, improve eye comfort, and support overall eye health.

Here are some effective techniques for stress reduction and relaxation:

Mindfulness Meditation: Mindfulness meditation involves focusing on the present moment without judgment. Practicing mindfulness can reduce stress and anxiety, helping to alleviate tension that may affect the eyes.

Deep Breathing Exercises: Deep breathing exercises help activate the body's relaxation response. Slow, deep breaths can calm the nervous system and reduce stress levels.

Progressive Muscle Relaxation: This technique involves systematically tensing and then relaxing different muscle groups in the body. Progressive muscle relaxation can help release physical tension and promote relaxation.

Yoga: Yoga combines physical postures, breathing exercises, and meditation to improve flexibility, balance, and overall well-being. Regular yoga practice can reduce stress and enhance eye comfort.

Tai Chi: Tai Chi is a gentle form of martial art that involves slow, flowing movements and deep breathing. It is known for promoting relaxation, reducing stress, and improving mind-body coordination.

Guided Imagery: Guided imagery involves visualizing calming and peaceful scenes, which can help reduce stress and promote relaxation.

Nature Walks: Spending time in nature, such as taking a walk in a park or a forest, can have a calming effect on the mind and reduce stress levels.

Listening to Music: Listening to soothing music can help relax the mind and alleviate stress.

Engaging in Hobbies: Participating in activities you enjoy, such as reading, painting, or gardening, can be a form of relaxation and stress reduction.

Social Support: Connecting with friends and loved ones, whether in person or virtually, can provide emotional support and help reduce stress.

Limiting Screen Time: Reducing screen time, especially before bedtime, can improve sleep quality and contribute to stress reduction.

Practicing Gratitude: Keeping a gratitude journal or reflecting on the positive aspects of your life can help shift focus away from stressors and promote a more positive outlook.

By incorporating these stress reduction techniques into your daily routine, you can enhance your ability to manage stress and improve overall eye comfort. Reducing stress not only benefits your eye health but also supports your overall physical and mental well-being. If you find it challenging to manage stress on your own, consider seeking professional guidance, such as counseling or therapy, to develop a personalized stress management plan. Remember that taking care of your overall health, including stress management, is essential for maintaining healthy and comfortable eyes.

CHAPTER 7: NATURAL REMEDIES AND HOME THERAPIES

In this chapter, we will explore natural remedies and home therapies that can provide relief from dry eye symptoms. From herbal remedies and natural treatments to DIY eye compresses and aromatherapy, these methods offer non-invasive and accessible options for managing dry eyes.

Herbal Remedies And Natural Treatments For Dry Eye

Herbal remedies and natural treatments offer alternative approaches for managing dry eye symptoms. While these remedies may not replace traditional medical treatments, some herbs and natural substances are believed to have properties that can alleviate dry eye discomfort and support overall eye health. Here are some herbal remedies and natural treatments for dry eye:

Omega-3 Fatty Acids: Omega-3 fatty acids are essential for maintaining a healthy tear film and reducing inflammation. Consuming foods rich in omega-3s, such as fatty fish (salmon, mackerel, sardines), chia seeds, flaxseeds, and walnuts, may help improve tear production and alleviate dry eye symptoms.

Bilberry Extract: Bilberry is a fruit related to blueberries and is known for its antioxidant properties. Some studies suggest that bilberry extract may have potential benefits for eye health, including supporting tear production and reducing eye fatigue.

Calendula: Calendula, also known as marigold, has anti-inflammatory properties and can be used as an eye wash or a compress to soothe irritated and dry eyes.

Chamomile: Chamomile has anti-inflammatory and calming properties that can be beneficial for eye health. Using chamomile tea bags as warm compresses or using chamomile-infused eye drops may help alleviate dry eye discomfort.

Green Tea: Green tea is rich in antioxidants and has anti-inflammatory effects. Applying cooled, damp green tea bags to closed eyes as compresses may provide relief from dry eye symptoms.

Aloe Vera: Aloe vera gel contains anti-inflammatory compounds and may help soothe irritated eyes. Applying a small amount of pure aloe vera gel to closed eyelids can provide a cooling and soothing effect.

Eyebright: Eyebright is an herb believed to have properties that can support eye health. It is available in various forms, such as eye drops or teas, and may help alleviate dry eye discomfort.

Ginkgo Biloba: Ginkgo biloba is an herb known for its antioxidant and anti-inflammatory properties. Some studies suggest that ginkgo biloba supplements may improve tear production and reduce dry eye symptoms.

Flaxseed Oil: Flaxseed oil is a source of omega-3 fatty acids and can be taken as a supplement to support tear production and overall eye health.

Before using any herbal remedies or natural treatments for dry eye, it is essential to consult with an eye care professional or a qualified healthcare provider. They can assess your specific eye health needs, provide personalized recommendations, and ensure that these remedies do not interact with any existing medications or conditions.

Additionally, herbal remedies should not be used as a sole treatment for severe or chronic dry eye conditions but can complement other dry eye management strategies for some individuals.

DIY Eye Compresses And Warm/Cold Therapy

DIY eye compresses and warm/cold therapy are simple yet effective home remedies that can provide relief from dry eye symptoms. These therapies can help soothe irritated eyes, improve tear film quality, and reduce inflammation. Here's how to create and use DIY eye compresses and warm/cold therapy for dry eye relief:

DIY Eye Compresses:

1. Warm Compress:
   - Soak a clean, soft cloth in warm water. Squeeze out excess water to avoid dripping.
   - Close your eyes and place the warm, damp cloth over your closed eyelids.
   - Keep the compress in place for 5 to 10 minutes, allowing the warmth to soothe and relax your eyes.

- Reheat the cloth as needed to maintain warmth during the session.

- The warm compress helps improve oil gland function along the eyelid margins, promoting better tear quality and eye lubrication.

2. Cold Compress:

- To create a cold compress, wrap a few ice cubes or a gel ice pack in a thin, clean cloth.

- Close your eyes and gently place the cold compress over your closed eyelids.

- Hold the compress in place for 5 to 10 minutes, taking breaks if it feels too cold.

- The cold compress helps reduce eye inflammation and soothes irritated eyes.

Warm/Cold Therapy:

1. Warm/Cold Contrast:

- For this therapy, start with a warm compress following the steps mentioned earlier.

- After using the warm compress, switch to a cold compress and apply it to your closed eyelids.

- Alternate between the warm and cold compresses for a few cycles, spending 5 to 10 minutes with each.

- The warm/cold contrast can help improve blood circulation around the eyes, reducing eye strain and relieving dry eye discomfort.

It's important to remember that DIY eye compresses and warm/cold therapy are intended for mild and occasional dry eye relief. If you experience persistent or severe dry eye symptoms, it's essential to consult with an eye care professional. They can assess your specific eye health needs, provide personalized recommendations, and address any underlying causes of your dry eye.

While these home therapies can be beneficial, they may not replace prescribed medications or medical treatments for chronic or severe dry eye conditions. Additionally, avoid applying excessive pressure to the eyes, and make sure the compresses are clean to avoid any risk of infection. With proper care and use, DIY eye compresses and warm/cold therapy can be valuable additions to your dry eye management routine, promoting more comfortable and healthier eyes.

Aromatherapy And Its Potential Benefits For Dry Eye Relief

Aromatherapy is a complementary therapy that uses aromatic essential oils derived from plants to promote physical and emotional well-being. While aromatherapy is not a substitute for medical treatment, some essential oils have potential benefits that may help alleviate dry eye symptoms and promote overall eye health. Here's how aromatherapy can be used for dry eye relief and its potential benefits:

Calming and Relaxing Effects: Aromatherapy with certain essential oils, such as lavender, chamomile, and rose, can have calming and relaxing effects on the mind and body. Stress and anxiety can contribute to dry eye symptoms, and using calming essential oils may help reduce tension and promote relaxation, potentially alleviating dry eye discomfort.

Anti-Inflammatory Properties: Some essential oils, like lavender and chamomile, possess anti-inflammatory properties that can help reduce eye inflammation associated with dry eye. Reducing inflammation may improve tear production and enhance eye comfort.

Soothing Irritated Eyes: Applying diluted chamomile or rose essential oils on a clean cloth and placing it over closed eyelids as a compress can help soothe irritated eyes. The gentle and cooling effect of these oils may provide relief from dry eye discomfort.

Promoting Better Sleep: Aromatherapy with lavender or vetiver essential oils may improve sleep quality. Adequate sleep is crucial for overall health, and getting enough rest can benefit eye health and reduce dry eye symptoms.

Supporting Tear Production: Some essential oils, such as rose and eucalyptus, are believed to have properties that can support tear production and improve tear film stability, promoting better eye moisture.

When Using Aromatherapy For Dry Eye Relief, It's Essential To Follow These Guidelines:

- Always dilute essential oils with a carrier oil (such as coconut or almond oil) before applying them to the skin or using them as compresses. Undiluted essential oils can cause skin irritation.
- Do not put essential oils directly into the eyes or apply them too close to the eye area.

- Conduct a patch test on a small area of skin to check for any allergic reactions or sensitivities before using essential oils for aromatherapy.
- Use high-quality, pure essential oils from reputable sources to ensure safety and efficacy.

It's important to note that individual responses to aromatherapy may vary, and some people may be sensitive to certain essential oils. If you have any existing eye conditions or allergies, consult with an eye care professional or a qualified healthcare provider before using aromatherapy for dry eye relief.

Aromatherapy can be a relaxing and enjoyable addition to your dry eye management routine. While it may provide some relief from dry eye discomfort, it is best used in combination with other dry eye treatments and lifestyle adjustments for more comprehensive care.

Chapter 8: Eye Care Products and Practices

In this chapter, we will explore essential eye care products and practices that are beneficial for managing dry eye symptoms. From evaluating eye drops and lubricants to selecting the right eye care products and considering appropriate eyewear, these tips will help improve eye comfort and support overall eye health. Here are the key topics covered in this chapter:

Evaluating Eye Drops And Lubricants For Dry Eye Management

Evaluating eye drops and lubricants is essential for effective dry eye management. With a wide range of products available, understanding their specific formulations and suitability for your dry eye condition is crucial. Here are some key factors to consider when evaluating eye drops and lubricants for dry eye management:

Type of Artificial Tears:
 - Artificial tears come in different types based on their viscosity and formulation. These include solutions, gels, and ointments.

- Solutions: Standard artificial tears are water-based and have a consistency similar to natural tears. They are suitable for mild to moderate dry eye symptoms and can be used frequently throughout the day.

- Gels: Gels have a thicker consistency than solutions and provide longer-lasting relief. They are ideal for moderate to severe dry eye symptoms and are often recommended for nighttime use due to their increased staying power on the ocular surface.

- Ointments: Ointments have the thickest consistency and provide the most prolonged relief. They are typically used at bedtime to help prevent dryness and discomfort during sleep.

Preservative-Free Options:

- Some artificial tears contain preservatives to prolong shelf life. However, frequent use of preserved eye drops may irritate the eyes, especially for individuals with sensitivity to preservatives.

- Preservative-free artificial tears are available in single-dose vials or unit-dose containers, and they are suitable for those who need to use eye drops frequently throughout the day or who have sensitivity to preservatives.

Specialized Formulas:

- Consider specialized eye drops that offer additional benefits beyond basic lubrication. Some formulations contain nutrients like omega-3 fatty acids, which can support overall eye health and reduce inflammation.

- Discuss with your eye care professional whether these specialized formulations are appropriate for your specific dry eye condition.

Compatibility with Contact Lenses:

- If you wear contact lenses, choose artificial tears that are compatible with your lens type. Some eye drops may be more suitable for contact lens wearers, while others can cause discomfort or interfere with lens performance.

Recommendations from an Eye Care Professional:

- Consult with an eye care professional, such as an optometrist or ophthalmologist, to determine the best eye drops or lubricants for your individual dry eye condition.

- Your eye care professional can assess the severity and underlying causes of your dry eye and recommend specific products tailored to your needs.

When evaluating eye drops and lubricants, it's essential to follow the recommended usage instructions provided on the product packaging. If you experience any adverse reactions or if your dry eye symptoms persist despite using eye drops, consult with your eye care professional for further evaluation and guidance. Remember that dry eye management may require a combination of strategies, including lifestyle adjustments, proper eye hygiene, and targeted treatments based on the underlying cause of your dry eye.

Tips For Selecting The Right Eye Care Products

Selecting the right eye care products is crucial for maintaining good eye health and managing specific eye conditions effectively. Whether you are looking for eye drops, contact lens solutions, or other eye care products, consider these tips to ensure you make the best choices for your individual needs:

Consult an Eye Care Professional: Before purchasing any eye care products, consult with an eye care professional, such as an optometrist or ophthalmologist. They can assess your eye health, identify any underlying issues, and provide personalized recommendations for the most suitable products.

Read Product Labels Carefully: Pay attention to the ingredients, usage instructions, and storage recommendations provided on the product labels. Avoid products with ingredients that may cause irritation or allergic reactions.

Look for Preservative-Free Options: If you have sensitive eyes or need to use eye drops frequently, consider choosing preservative-free eye drops. These are available in single-dose vials or unit-dose containers and can reduce the risk of irritation associated with preservatives.

Choose High-Quality Products: Opt for eye care products from reputable brands and sources. High-quality products are more likely to meet safety standards and provide effective results.

Consider Your Eye Condition: Different eye conditions may require specific products. For example, if you have dry eyes, you may need lubricating eye drops or gels, while individuals with allergies might benefit from antihistamine eye drops.

Compatibility with Contact Lenses: If you wear contact lenses, ensure that the eye care products you use are compatible with your specific lens type. Some solutions may be designed for soft lenses, while others are intended for rigid gas permeable lenses.

Check Expiry Dates: Always check the expiry dates of eye care products before use. Using expired products can lead to reduced effectiveness or potential risks.

Avoid Sharing Products: To prevent the spread of eye infections, avoid sharing eye care products with others.

Monitor Any Adverse Reactions: If you experience any discomfort, irritation, or adverse reactions after using an eye care product, discontinue use and consult your eye care professional.

Follow Recommended Dosage: Use eye care products as directed by your eye care professional or according to the instructions provided on the product packaging. Using more than the recommended dosage may not provide additional benefits and can lead to unwanted side effects.

Store Properly: Follow storage instructions for eye care products. Some products may need to be stored in a cool, dry place, while others may require refrigeration.

Remember that individual responses to eye care products may vary, and what works well for one person may not work for another. If you have any concerns or questions about selecting the right eye care products, do not hesitate to seek guidance from your eye care professional. Taking a proactive approach to eye care and using appropriate products can contribute to maintaining healthy and comfortable eyes.

Eyewear Considerations For Dry Eye Sufferers

Eyewear considerations are crucial for dry eye sufferers to minimize eye strain, protect the eyes from environmental irritants, and maintain better eye moisture. Here are some key factors to consider when choosing eyewear for individuals with dry eyes:

Moisture Chamber Glasses:
  - Moisture chamber glasses create a protective barrier around the eyes, reducing the rate of tear evaporation and maintaining eye moisture.
  - These glasses are particularly beneficial for individuals with evaporative dry eye, where tears evaporate too quickly from the ocular surface.

Wraparound Sunglasses:

- Wraparound sunglasses offer additional coverage, shielding the eyes from wind, dust, and other environmental irritants that can exacerbate dry eye symptoms.

- These sunglasses are especially helpful in windy or dusty environments, providing extra protection and reducing eye discomfort.

Computer Glasses:

- Computer glasses with an anti-glare coating can help reduce eye strain during prolonged screen use.

- These glasses are designed to filter out harmful blue light emitted by digital screens, which can contribute to eye fatigue and dryness.

Prescription Eyewear Considerations:

- If you wear prescription glasses, discuss with your optometrist or ophthalmologist the possibility of incorporating specific coatings or treatments to improve eye comfort.

- Options may include anti-reflective coatings to minimize glare and reduce eye strain, or lens materials designed to retain moisture.

Proper Fit and Comfort:

- Ensure that any eyewear you choose fits well and is comfortable to wear for extended periods.

- Ill-fitting glasses may cause additional irritation or discomfort, so it's essential to find the right frame size and style that suits your needs.

Keep Lenses Clean:

- Regularly clean your eyewear lenses to remove dust, debris, or other particles that can contribute to eye irritation.

- Clean lenses provide better clarity and reduce the risk of eye strain.

Use Eyewear Consistently:

- Incorporate the appropriate eyewear into your daily routine consistently, especially in situations where it can protect your eyes from dry air, wind, or glare.

Remember that while eyewear considerations can help alleviate dry eye symptoms, they should not replace other dry eye management strategies or professional treatment. It's crucial to consult with an eye care professional to assess the severity and underlying causes of your dry eye and receive tailored recommendations for managing your condition.

In addition to wearing appropriate eyewear, practicing good eye hygiene, using prescribed eye drops or lubricants as directed, and making lifestyle adjustments can significantly contribute to better eye comfort and overall eye health for dry eye sufferers.

CHAPTER 9: BEYOND THE BASICS: ADVANCED DRY EYE SOLUTIONS

In this chapter, we will explore advanced dry eye solutions that go beyond traditional approaches. These advanced strategies leverage cutting-edge research and integrative medicine to provide relief for severe dry eye cases.

The Role Of Omega-3 Fatty Acids In Dry Rye Management

Omega-3 fatty acids play a significant role in dry eye management and overall eye health. These essential fatty acids, particularly eicosapentaenoic acid (EPA) and docosahexaenoic acid (DHA), are crucial components of cell membranes and are abundant in the retina and other eye tissues. Here are the key ways in which omega-3 fatty acids contribute to dry eye management:

Anti-Inflammatory Properties: Omega-3 fatty acids have potent anti-inflammatory effects. Inflammation is a common underlying factor in dry eye, especially in cases of evaporative dry eye, where there is dysfunction of the meibomian glands that produce the lipid layer of tears. By reducing ocular surface inflammation, omega-3s can help improve tear film stability and reduce dry eye symptoms.

Improving Tear Film Quality: The lipid layer of the tear film is essential for preventing excessive tear evaporation. Omega-3 fatty acids help enhance the composition of this lipid layer, making it more resistant to evaporation. This improvement in tear film quality leads to better eye moisture and reduced dryness.

Stimulating Tear Production: Omega-3 fatty acids may support lacrimal gland function, the glands responsible for producing the aqueous layer of tears. By promoting tear production, omega-3s contribute to maintaining adequate eye lubrication and comfort.

Antioxidant Properties: Omega-3s have antioxidant properties, which help protect the eyes from oxidative stress caused by free radicals. Oxidative stress can damage eye tissues and exacerbate dry eye symptoms. Antioxidants neutralize free radicals, reducing their harmful effects on the eyes.

Modulating Immune Responses: Omega-3s can influence immune responses in the body, helping to regulate the immune system's activity and prevent excessive inflammation in the eyes. This immune modulation can be beneficial for individuals with autoimmune-related dry eye conditions.

To incorporate omega-3 fatty acids into your dry eye management, consider the following sources:

- Fatty Fish: Fish like salmon, mackerel, sardines, and trout are excellent sources of EPA and DHA.
- Plant-Based Sources: Flaxseeds, chia seeds, and walnuts are rich in alpha-linolenic acid (ALA), a type of omega-3 fatty acid that the body can convert into EPA and DHA to a limited extent.
- Supplements: Omega-3 supplements, such as fish oil capsules or algae-based supplements for those following a vegetarian or vegan diet, can be used to ensure adequate intake.

Before starting any supplements, it's essential to consult with an eye care professional or a qualified healthcare provider, especially if you have any existing medical conditions or are taking medications. They can provide personalized recommendations and guidance on the appropriate dosage to meet your specific needs.

Incorporating omega-3 fatty acids into your diet or as supplements, in conjunction with other dry eye management strategies, can contribute to better eye comfort and support overall eye health.

Integrative Medicine And Its Potential For Dry Eye Relief

Integrative medicine offers a holistic approach to dry eye relief, combining conventional medical treatments with complementary therapies to address not only the physical symptoms but also the emotional and psychological aspects of the condition. Integrative medicine recognizes the interconnectedness of various factors that can influence dry eye, such as stress, diet, lifestyle, and overall health. Here are some ways in which integrative medicine can potentially provide dry eye relief:

Mind-Body Connection: Integrative medicine emphasizes the mind-body connection and acknowledges that stress and emotional well-being can impact physical health, including eye health. Stress can exacerbate dry eye symptoms and contribute to eye strain. Techniques like mindfulness-based stress reduction, meditation, and deep breathing exercises are used in integrative medicine to help manage stress and promote relaxation, potentially reducing dry eye discomfort.

Acupuncture: Acupuncture is an ancient Chinese therapy that involves the insertion of thin needles into specific points on the body. Some studies suggest that acupuncture may have benefits for dry eye by improving tear production and reducing inflammation. It is believed to help balance the body's energy (qi) and promote overall well-being.

Nutrition and Supplements: Integrative medicine encourages a balanced and nutrient-rich diet to support overall health, including eye health. Certain nutrients, such as omega-3 fatty acids, vitamin A, and antioxidants, have been linked to better tear production and eye moisture. Integrative practitioners may recommend specific dietary changes or supplements to address nutritional deficiencies and promote eye health.

Herbal Remedies: Herbal remedies are commonly used in integrative medicine for various health conditions, including dry eye. Some herbs, such as calendula and chamomile, have anti-inflammatory properties and can be used as eye compresses or washes to soothe irritated eyes.

Lifestyle Modifications: Integrative medicine emphasizes the importance of lifestyle adjustments to support eye health. This may include optimizing sleep, reducing screen time, maintaining proper hydration, and managing environmental factors that can contribute to dry eye symptoms.

Collaborative Care: Integrative medicine encourages collaboration between different healthcare providers to develop a comprehensive treatment plan. This may involve working with an eye care professional, a nutritionist, a stress management specialist, and other practitioners to address the various aspects of dry eye.

While integrative medicine can offer additional strategies for dry eye relief, it's essential to work with qualified practitioners who have expertise in both conventional and complementary approaches. Before incorporating any complementary therapies or supplements, consult with an eye care professional or a qualified healthcare provider to ensure they are safe and appropriate for your specific dry eye condition.

Integrative medicine can complement conventional dry eye treatments and provide a more personalized and comprehensive approach to managing dry eye symptoms. By addressing the root causes of dry eye and promoting overall well-being, integrative medicine may help individuals find relief and improve their quality of life.

New And Emerging Treatments For Severe Dry Eye Cases

New and emerging treatments for severe dry eye cases are continually being researched and developed to provide more effective and targeted solutions for individuals who do not find adequate relief with conventional therapies. These innovative treatments aim to address the underlying causes of severe dry eye and improve tear production and quality. Here are some of the promising new and emerging treatments for severe dry eye:

Regenerative Medicine Therapies:
 - Autologous Serum Eye Drops: Autologous serum eye drops are made from a patient's own blood serum, which contains essential growth factors and nutrients. These drops can help promote healing and reduce inflammation on the ocular surface, providing relief for severe dry eye cases.
 - Amniotic Membrane Transplantation: Amniotic membrane transplantation involves the placement of an

amniotic membrane graft on the ocular surface. This technique can help reduce inflammation, support tissue healing, and improve tear film stability in severe dry eye cases.

Tear Stimulating Therapies:

- Neurostimulation Devices: Neurostimulation devices are designed to stimulate the nerves responsible for tear production. These devices use gentle electrical impulses to trigger tear production, offering an alternative option for individuals with severe dry eye resistant to other treatments.
- Punctal Plugs and Occluders: Punctal plugs and occluders are small devices inserted into the tear drainage ducts to slow down the drainage of tears from the eyes. This helps to retain more tears on the ocular surface, providing increased moisture and relief for severe dry eye.

Cytokine Modulators:

- Cytokine modulators are medications that target specific inflammatory molecules involved in the development of dry eye. By blocking or inhibiting these molecules, cytokine modulators can reduce ocular surface inflammation and improve tear film stability.

Lipid-Based Therapies:

- Lipid-based therapies focus on improving the quality and composition of the lipid layer of the tear film. New formulations of lipid-based eye drops and ointments aim to enhance the protective function of the lipid layer and reduce tear evaporation.

Biologic Therapies:
- Biologic therapies involve the use of targeted biological agents to address specific inflammatory pathways involved in dry eye. These therapies can modulate the immune response and reduce ocular surface inflammation.

It's important to note that while these new and emerging treatments show promising results, they are often still in the research and development stages or may have limited availability. Additionally, not all treatments are suitable for every individual with severe dry eye, and some may require further investigation to determine their long-term efficacy and safety.

Individuals with severe dry eye should work closely with their eye care professional or a dry eye specialist to explore the most appropriate treatment options based on their specific condition and needs. As research progresses, more effective and targeted treatments for severe dry eye are likely to become available, offering hope for improved eye comfort and quality of life for those who are affected by this challenging condition.

CHAPTER 10: PREVENTION AND LONG-TERM MAINTENANCE

In this chapter, we focus on prevention strategies and long-term maintenance for dry eye management. It's essential to implement proactive measures to prevent dry eye from worsening and to create a comprehensive plan for maintaining eye health and comfort over the long term.

Strategies For Preventing Dry Eye From Worsening

Strategies for preventing dry eye from worsening are essential for maintaining eye comfort and overall eye health. Implementing proactive measures can help reduce the severity of dry eye symptoms and prevent further complications. Here are some effective strategies to prevent dry eye from worsening:

Maintain Adequate Hydration: Drink plenty of water throughout the day to stay well-hydrated. Proper hydration supports tear production and helps maintain eye moisture.

Follow the 20-20-20 Rule: During visually intensive tasks, such as using a computer or reading, take breaks every 20 minutes. Look at something 20 feet away for at least 20 seconds. This practice helps reduce eye strain and supports a healthy tear film.

Blink Regularly: Consciously blink your eyes regularly, especially during extended screen time or other activities that may cause decreased blinking. Blinking spreads tears across the ocular surface, keeping your eyes moist.

Use Humidifiers: In dry indoor environments, especially during the winter months, use humidifiers to add moisture to the air. Humidifiers can help prevent excessive tear evaporation.

Protect Your Eyes: Wear wraparound sunglasses or protective eyewear when exposed to wind, dust, or other environmental irritants that can exacerbate dry eye symptoms.

Adjust Computer Screen Settings: Position your computer screen slightly below eye level and reduce screen glare to reduce eye strain during prolonged computer use.

Maintain Proper Eyelid Hygiene: Practice good eyelid hygiene by gently cleaning the eyelids and lashes daily to prevent blockage of the meibomian glands and reduce the risk of meibomian gland dysfunction.

Avoid Smoke and Irritants: Avoid smoking and exposure to secondhand smoke, as well as other environmental irritants that can worsen dry eye symptoms.

Consider Nutritional Support: Consume a balanced diet rich in omega-3 fatty acids, antioxidants, and vitamins that support eye health. Omega-3s, in particular, have been linked to improved tear production and quality.

Limit Eye Strain: Use proper lighting when reading or working on the computer to reduce eye strain. Adjust the brightness and contrast settings on screens to a comfortable level.

Manage Chronic Health Conditions: If you have underlying health conditions, such as diabetes, autoimmune disorders, or hormonal imbalances, work with your healthcare provider to manage them effectively, as these conditions can contribute to dry eye.

Regular Eye Checkups: Schedule regular comprehensive eye exams with an eye care professional to monitor your eye health, identify any changes in your dry eye condition, and adjust your treatment plan accordingly.

By incorporating these preventive strategies into your daily routine, you can reduce the risk of dry eye worsening and enjoy better eye comfort and health. If you experience persistent or severe dry eye symptoms, consult with an eye care professional for a thorough evaluation and personalized recommendations. Early intervention and consistent eye care can make a significant difference in managing dry eye effectively.

Creating A Long-Term Plan For Eye Health And Comfort

Creating a long-term plan for eye health and comfort involves developing sustainable habits and incorporating preventive measures to support your eyes' well-being throughout your life. By adopting a proactive approach to eye care, you can minimize the risk of eye discomfort, reduce the impact of potential eye conditions, and maintain clear vision. Here are the key components to consider when creating a long-term plan for eye health and comfort:

Comprehensive Eye Exams:

- Schedule regular comprehensive eye exams with an eye care professional, such as an optometrist or ophthalmologist.

- These exams allow for early detection of eye conditions, including dry eye, and prompt intervention to prevent progression and potential complications.

Lifestyle Adjustments:

- Make lifestyle adjustments that promote eye health, such as reducing screen time, taking breaks during visually intensive tasks, and avoiding excessive eye strain.

- Incorporate regular physical activity into your routine to support overall health, which can indirectly benefit your eyes.

Proper Hydration:

- Stay well-hydrated by drinking an adequate amount of water daily.

- Proper hydration supports tear production and helps maintain eye moisture, preventing dry eye symptoms.

Eye-Friendly Nutrition:

- Consume a balanced diet rich in nutrients that support eye health, such as omega-3 fatty acids, vitamins A, C, and E, and antioxidants.

- Consider incorporating foods like fatty fish, leafy greens, citrus fruits, and nuts into your diet.

Protect Your Eyes:

- Wear appropriate eyewear, such as sunglasses with UV protection, when outdoors to shield your eyes from harmful ultraviolet rays.

- Consider wearing protective eyewear when engaging in sports or activities that could pose a risk of eye injury.

Regular Eye Hygiene:

- Practice good eye hygiene by washing your hands before touching your eyes and using a clean cloth for wiping your face.

- Cleanse your eyelids and eyelashes gently to prevent blockage of the meibomian glands and reduce the risk of eye irritation.

Proper Computer Use:

- Position your computer screen at eye level and maintain a comfortable distance to reduce eye strain.

- Follow the 20-20-20 rule: Take breaks every 20 minutes, look at something 20 feet away, and blink for 20 seconds to prevent eye fatigue during prolonged screen use.

Limit Environmental Irritants:

- Avoid exposure to smoke and other irritants that can worsen dry eye symptoms.

- Use humidifiers to add moisture to dry indoor environments, especially during the winter months.

Collaborate with Eye Care Professionals:

- Work closely with your eye care professional to develop a personalized long-term plan for eye health and comfort.

- Regularly update them about any changes or concerns related to your eye health.

A well-rounded and consistent long-term plan for eye health and comfort can contribute to clear vision and reduce the risk of developing eye conditions or complications. Be proactive about your eye care and implement these strategies into your daily life to ensure that your eyes remain healthy and comfortable throughout the years. Remember that every individual's eye health is unique, so it's essential to work closely with your eye care professional to tailor the plan to your specific needs and circumstances.

Regular Eye Checkups And Their Importance For Dry Eye Management

Regular eye checkups are essential for effective dry eye management as they play a crucial role in monitoring the condition, identifying any changes or progression, and adjusting the treatment plan accordingly. Here are the key reasons why regular eye checkups are important for dry eye management:

Early Detection and Diagnosis: Regular eye exams allow for the early detection and diagnosis of dry eye. Dry eye symptoms can be subtle and easily overlooked, especially in the early stages. During an eye checkup, an eye care professional can assess your tear film quality, tear production, and the health of your ocular surface, enabling early intervention if dry eye is detected.

Personalized Treatment Plan: An eye care professional can develop a personalized treatment plan based on the severity and underlying causes of your dry eye. This tailored approach is crucial as different individuals may experience dry eye due to various factors, such as meibomian gland dysfunction, tear deficiency, or inflammatory conditions.

Monitoring Progression: Regular eye checkups allow your eye care professional to monitor the progression of your dry eye over time. This helps to determine if the current treatment is effective or if adjustments are necessary to manage changing symptoms.

Adjustment of Treatment: If your dry eye symptoms change or worsen, your eye care professional can adjust your treatment plan accordingly. This may involve modifying the type of eye drops or lubricants you use, recommending additional therapies, or addressing new underlying factors contributing to your dry eye.

Managing Underlying Conditions: Dry eye can be associated with various underlying health conditions, such as autoimmune disorders, hormonal imbalances, or allergies. Regular eye exams can help identify these conditions, allowing for timely management and preventing their exacerbation of dry eye symptoms.

Education and Support: Eye care professionals can educate you about proper eye hygiene, lifestyle modifications, and environmental adjustments to manage dry eye effectively between checkups. They can also provide support and guidance throughout your dry eye management journey.

Prevention of Complications: Unmanaged dry eye can lead to complications, such as corneal damage or increased risk of eye infections. Regular eye checkups help prevent such complications by detecting and managing dry eye early.

Identification of New Treatments: As new treatments and therapies for dry eye emerge, your eye care professional can inform you about these advancements and discuss whether they may be suitable for your condition.

Overall, regular eye checkups are crucial for managing dry eye and maintaining eye health. They empower you to take a proactive approach to your eye care, receive appropriate treatment and support, and prevent potential complications. Be sure to schedule routine eye exams as recommended by your eye care professional, even if you are not experiencing noticeable dry eye symptoms, to ensure that your eyes remain healthy and comfortable.

CHAPTER 11: EMBRACING THE REFRESH: YOUR PERSONAL DRY EYE ACTION PLAN

In this final chapter, we bring all the knowledge and strategies discussed throughout the book together to create your personalized dry eye action plan. This comprehensive plan will help you effectively manage dry eye, set achievable goals, and track your progress. By embracing a holistic approach to lifelong eye health, you can enjoy lasting relief and maintain optimal eye comfort. Here are the key elements of your personalized dry eye action plan:

Understanding Your Dry Eye:

- Review the chapters on dry eye causes, symptoms, and different types to gain a comprehensive understanding of your condition.

Lifestyle and Environmental Adjustments:

- Implement lifestyle changes and environmental adjustments that support eye health and minimize dry eye symptoms, such as practicing the 20-20-20 rule, using humidifiers, and protecting your eyes from irritants.

Nutritional Support:

- Include eye-friendly foods rich in omega-3 fatty acids, antioxidants, and vitamins in your diet to support tear production and overall eye health.

Proper Hydration:

- Stay well-hydrated by drinking an adequate amount of water throughout the day to promote tear production and reduce dry eye discomfort.

Eye Hygiene:

- Practice good eye hygiene by keeping your eyelids and eyelashes clean to prevent meibomian gland dysfunction and eye irritation.

Medications and Therapies:

- Follow your eye care professional's recommendations for prescribed eye drops, lubricants, or other therapies to manage your dry eye condition effectively.

Holistic Practices:

- Embrace stress reduction techniques, such as mindfulness, meditation, or yoga, to address the mind-body connection and promote overall well-being.

Goal Setting and Tracking Progress:

- Set specific, achievable goals for your dry eye management, such as reducing eye discomfort during screen time or maintaining a certain level of eye moisture.

- Track your progress regularly and make adjustments to your action plan as needed to keep moving towards your goals.

Regular Eye Checkups:

- Schedule routine comprehensive eye exams with your eye care professional to monitor your dry eye condition, adjust your treatment plan, and address any underlying health conditions.

Lifelong Eye Health:

- Embrace a holistic approach to lifelong eye health by integrating your dry eye action plan into your daily routine, making it a part of your overall wellness journey.

By creating and implementing your personalized dry eye action plan, you take control of your eye health and embrace the refreshment of lasting eye comfort. Remember that each individual's dry eye condition is unique, so your action plan should be tailored to your specific needs and circumstances.

Continue to work closely with your eye care professional to receive ongoing support and guidance as you progress on your dry eye management journey. With consistent care and a holistic approach, you can enjoy better eye comfort, protect your eye health, and embrace a refreshing outlook on lifelong eye care.

CONCLUSION

As we reach the end of "Embrace the Refresh: A Holistic Approach to Dry Eye Solutions," we stand at the threshold of a transformative journey towards lasting relief, eye health, and overall well-being. Throughout these pages, we have explored the intricate world of dry eye, uncovering the multifaceted factors that contribute to this common but often misunderstood condition.

From understanding the nuances of dry eye syndrome to recognizing the impact of lifestyle, nutrition, and stress on our ocular comfort, we have discovered the power of a holistic approach to eye care. By embracing the interconnectedness of our physical, emotional, and environmental well-being, we have empowered ourselves to become stewards of our own eye health.

We have explored the wonders of nutrition, discovering eye-friendly foods and supplements that nourish our eyes from within. Our journey has taken us on an exploration of herbal remedies, compresses, and aromatherapy, finding solace in nature's gifts for dry eye relief.

But perhaps most importantly, we have embraced the profound connection between our mind and body, understanding that stress and emotional well-being play a pivotal role in the health of our eyes. By incorporating stress reduction techniques, lifestyle adjustments, and mindfulness practices into our daily lives, we have harnessed the power of holistic healing.

We have developed personalized dry eye action plans, setting goals and tracking progress, ensuring that our journey towards relief and rejuvenation is guided by purpose and intention. Our action plans have become blueprints for lifelong eye health, perpetuating the refreshment and comfort that we seek.

As we conclude this journey, we invite you to carry the wisdom of these pages into your daily life. Embrace the refreshment that comes from taking charge of your eye health and nourishing your body, mind, and soul. Recognize the significance of the small changes that can make a significant impact on your ocular comfort and overall well-being.

Let "Embrace the Refresh" be a constant reminder that our eyes are precious gifts, deserving of tender care and compassion. As we continue on our life's path, let us remember that self-care and rejuvenation are not fleeting pursuits but lifelong commitments to our well-being.

May this book serve as a guiding light on your journey towards eye health and comfort. As you embrace the refreshment of a holistic approach, may your eyes sparkle with vitality, and may you find lasting relief and joy in the simple act of caring for your precious eyes.

Thank you for joining us on this transformative journey. Let us move forward, empowered by knowledge, nourished by compassion, and refreshed by the beauty of lifelong eye health.

With refreshed eyes and hearts, we bid you farewell until we meet again.

Embrace the refreshment, embrace your eye health, and embrace life's vibrant perspectives.

Wishing you a life filled with comfort, clarity, and the joy of embracing the refreshment of your eyes.

Goodbye, And Take Care.

www.ingramcontent.com/pod-product-compliance
Lightning Source LLC
Chambersburg PA
CBHW070953250726
48663CB00002B/198